Rim Khemakhem
Rahma Gargouri
Nedia Moussa

Smoking cessation

Rim Khemakhem
Rahma Gargouri
Nedia Moussa

Smoking cessation

Smoking and hospitalization of a loved one: the decisive influence on quitting smoking

ScienciaScripts

Imprint

Any brand names and product names mentioned in this book are subject to trademark, brand or patent protection and are trademarks or registered trademarks of their respective holders. The use of brand names, product names, common names, trade names, product descriptions etc. even without a particular marking in this work is in no way to be construed to mean that such names may be regarded as unrestricted in respect of trademark and brand protection legislation and could thus be used by anyone.

Cover image: www.ingimage.com

This book is a translation from the original published under ISBN 978-620-6-70812-4.

Publisher:
Sciencia Scripts
is a trademark of
Dodo Books Indian Ocean Ltd. and OmniScriptum S.R.L publishing group

120 High Road, East Finchley, London, N2 9ED, United Kingdom
Str. Armeneasca 28/1, office 1, Chisinau MD-2012, Republic of Moldova, Europe
Printed at: see last page
ISBN: 978-620-7-85411-0

CONTENTS

List of abbreviations

COPD: Chronic obstructive pulmonary disease

CBP: Bronchopulmonary cancer

COE: Carbon monoxide in exhaled air

DDB: bronchial dilatation

PE: Pulmonary embolism

HAD: Hospital Anxiety Depression

HBSC: Health behaviour in school-aged children

WHO: World Health Organization

PNO: Pneumothorax

SAS: Sleep apnea syndrome

CBT: Cognitive behavioral therapy

Introduction

Smoking is one of the main risk factors for many chronic diseases, such as cancer, lung disease and cardiovascular disease.

Every year, it is responsible for over 6 million deaths worldwide and almost 80,000 in France, and could be responsible for 1 billion deaths in the 21st century (1-3).

Weaning aid is the fundamental step in the treatment process. It is considered to be one of the most effective ways of contributing to a one-third reduction in premature mortality from non-communicable diseases worldwide by 2030(4).

However, smoking induces dependency, which makes weaning difficult.

Several studies have highlighted the need to complement collective measures with individual care, particularly for the most dependent smokers (5, 6,7). Improving the effectiveness of smoking cessation aid requires filling the gaps in our knowledge of tobacco dependence and the factors influencing motivation to stop smoking. To advance research, studies are needed not only on the therapeutic efficacy of cessation aid methods, but also on the social or psychological determinants influencing motivation to quit smoking(7, 8).

With this in mind, we conducted this study among smokers who had a loved one hospitalized in the pneumology department in order to..:

1. Study the particularities of smoking in these subjects.

2. Define the frequency of mood disorders in them.

3. Evaluate the impact of a loved one's hospitalization on their motivation to quit smoking.

Materials and methods

1. TYPE OF STUDY:

We conducted a cross-sectional study, including smoking subjects visiting a loved one hospitalized in the pneumology department of CHU Hédi Chakerde Sfax for 2 months (running from April to May 2018).

2. METHODOLOGY:

- ✓ Based on a questionnaire, the following data were collected:

  - Age

  - Comorbidities

  - Co-addictions

  - Smoking characteristics: type of tobacco, duration of smoking, daily tobacco consumption, age of first cigarette.

  - Withdrawal attempts: defined by a previous withdrawal of more than 7 days.

  - Physical dependence assessed by the Fagerstrom test (9).

  - Motivation to quit smoking assessed by the Quit Motivation Questionnaire (Q-MAT) (motivation defined as good if score > 13)(10).

  - Anxiety-depressive state identified by the Hospital Anxiety Depression (HAD) test with its Arabic version(11).

- ✓ Smokers surveyed were contacted by telephone after 3 months to reassess their smoking status.

1. 3. statistical analysis:

The statistical study was carried out using SPSS 20 software, with qualitative variables being compared using the Chi 2 test and quantitative variables using the Student test. The threshold of statistical significance was set at 5%, and the Chi 2 test was used for the comparative study of qualitative variables, and the Fischer (P) test for small samples.

Results

1. EPIDEMIOLOGICAL DATA:

Seventy (70) subjects completed the questionnaires.

1.1. Gender and age:

All subjects were male.

The mean age was 40± 15.2 years, with extremes ranging from 15 to 76 years.

1.2. Socioeconomic level:

The subjects studied were of urban origin in 74% of cases.

Fifty percent of subjects had a primary school education (Figure 1).

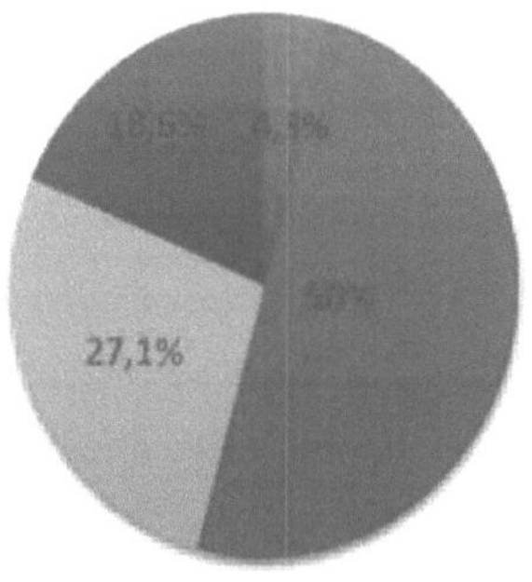

__Figure 1: Distribution of smokers by intellectual level__[di].

2. PERSONAL ANTECEDENTS OF SURVEYED SMOKERS:

None of the subjects had a history of respiratory pathology.

3. REASONS FOR HOSPITALIZATION OF RELATIVES:

The most common reasons for hospitalization were decompensation of chronic obstructive pulmonary disease (COPD) (36.5%) and bronchopulmonary cancer (PBC) (27%) (Table I).

Table I: Reasons for hospitalization of relatives

Pathology	Percentage (%)
COPD decompensation	36,5
Bronchopulmonary cancer	27,0
Bronchial dilatation	7,9
Asthma	6,3
Pleuresis	6,3
Pulmonary embolism	6,3
Sleep apnea syndrome	6,3
Pneumothorax	3,2

4. CHARACTERISTICS OF SMOKING:

4.1. Type of smoking:

Cigarettes were the most commonly used type of tobacco (97% of cases).

Hookah is a mode of consumption that appeals to 2.9% of the population (Figure 2).

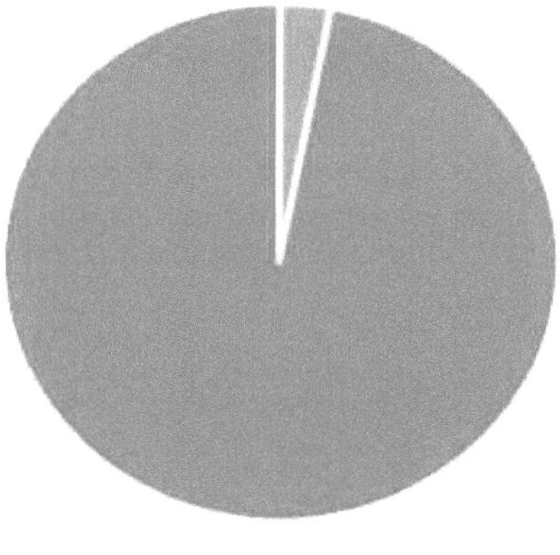

Figure 2: Type of tobacco used[d2].

4.2. Age of first consumption:

The average age of first smoking was 17, with extremes ranging from 8 to 35 years.

A significant difference was noted between age of first cigarette and different socioeconomic levels (p=0.042). The lower the socioeconomic level, the younger the age of first smoking.

4.3. Average tobacco consumption:

All subjects had people around them who smoked.

Average consumption was 28PA, with 77% smoking more than 10 PA and 28% more than 30 PA (figure n°3).

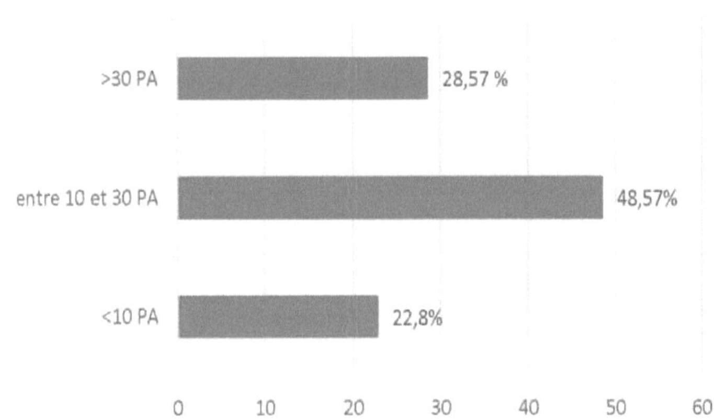

Figure 3: Distribution of smokers according to tobacco consumption in pack-years (PA[d3]*/*

Tobacco consumption was higher among subjects with a lower socio-economic and intellectual level (p=0.040) (figure 4). However, no significant difference was found between tobacco consumption and urban or rural origin (p=0.54).

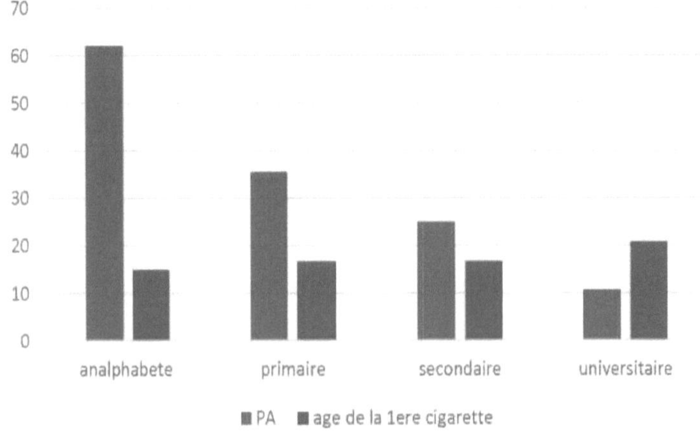

Figure 4: Tobacco consumption by socio-economic and intellectual level

4.4. Consumption time:

The average duration of smoking was 22 years, with extremes ranging from 2 to 66 years.

5. CO-ADDICTIONS:

Alcoholism was noted in 22.7% of smokers.

6. EVALUATION OF TOBACCO DEPENDENCE:

Dependence was judged as high (35.7%), medium (18.6%), low (20%) and absent (25.7%) (Figure n°5[d4]).

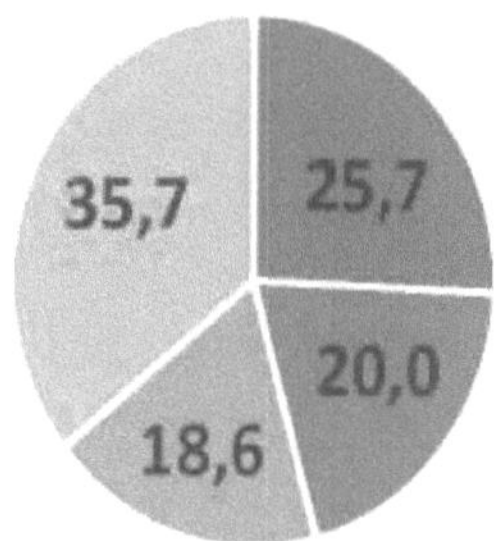

Figure 5: Distribution of smokers by level of tobacco dependence

There was an association between age of first cigarette (p=0.02), number of APs (p=0.04) and tobacco dependence. It seems that the younger the age of first smoking, the greater the number of APs and the stronger the dependence.

7. PSYCHOLOGICAL PROFILE OF SURVEYED SMOKERS:

7.1. Anxiety-depressive disorders:

An anxiety disorder was noted in 41.4% of subjects, and a depressive disorder in 11.4% (Figure 6).

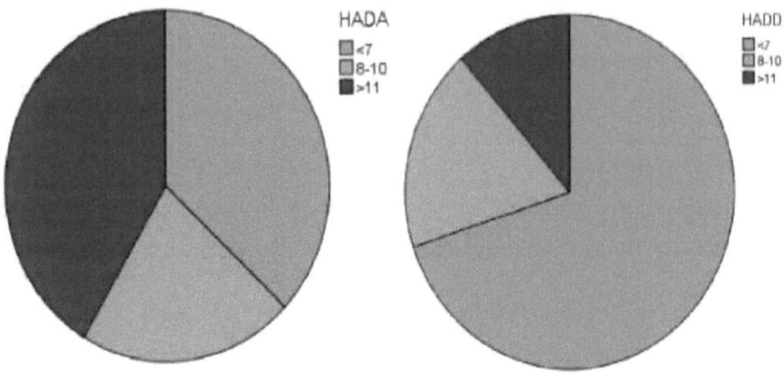

Figure 6: Anxiety-depressive disorders in surveyed smokers

HADA*: HAD score for anxiety; HADD*: HAD score for depression

7.2. Correlation between anxiety-depressive disorders and pathology of hospitalized family member

No correlation was found between <u>depressive disorders</u> and socioeconomic level (p=0.13) or cause of hospitalization of the relative (p=0.57).

In addition, a positive association was noted between <u>anxiety disorders</u> and the cause of the parent's hospitalization.

Indeed, subjects who had a relative hospitalized for a smoking-related pathology (chronic obstructive pulmonary disease, bronchopulmonary cancer) tended to have an anxiety disorder (figure n°7).

Of the subjects surveyed with anxiety disorders, 44% had a close relative hospitalized for COPD decompensation, and 36.6% had a close relative being followed for PBC. Similarly, these subjects appear to have a shorter average smoking duration (17.67±9.94 versus 29.32±17.4 years).

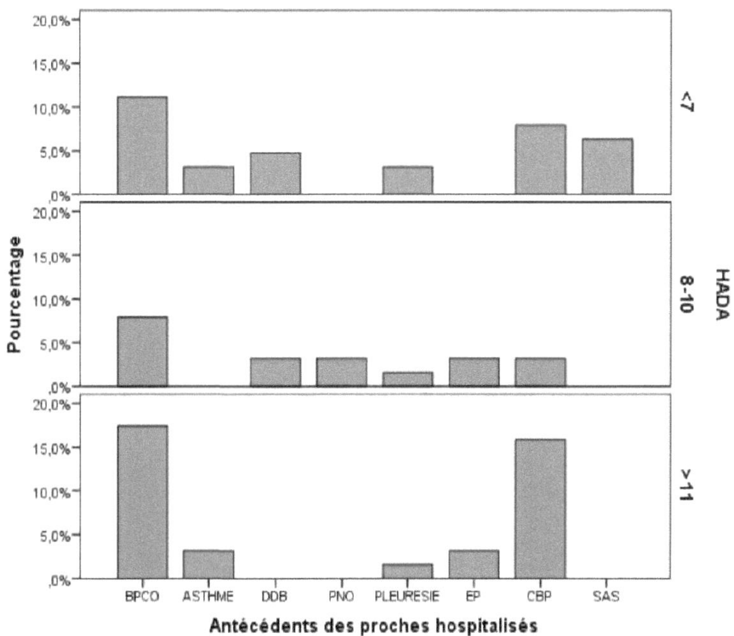

<u>Figure 7: Distribution of the pathology of the hospitalised relative according to the anxiety disorder of smokers.</u>

DDB*: bronchial dilatation; PNO*: pneumothorax; PE*: pulmonary embolism; CBP*: bronchopulmonary cancer; SAS*: sleep apnea syndrome

8. MOTIVATION TO STOP SMOKING:

8.1. Weaning attempts:

Previous quit attempts were reported by 21% of subjects.

The number of quit attempts was one (11.4%), 2 (4.3%) and 3 (2.9%) (Figure 8).

None of the patients used medication (Nico patch or nicopass) or cognitive-behavioral therapy.

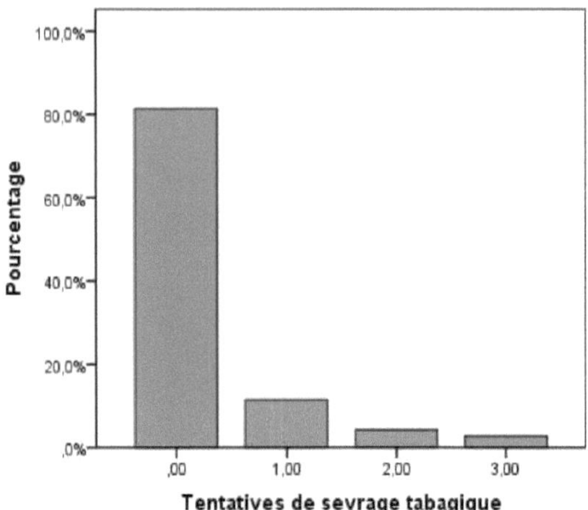

Figure 8: Number of quit attempts among smokers

8.2. Assessment of motivation to stop smoking:

Very good motivation to quit smoking was found in 32.9% of cases (Figure 9).

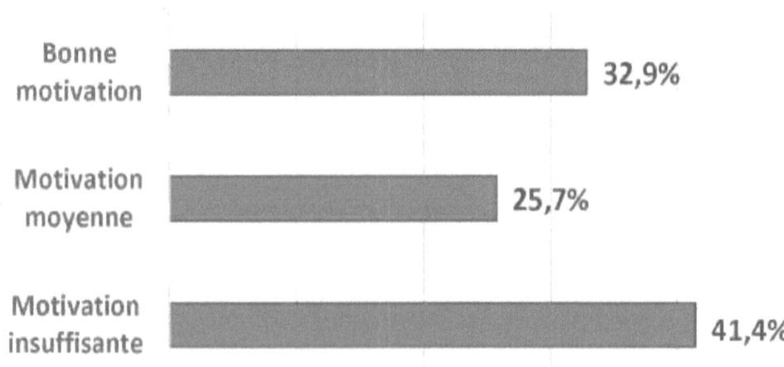

Figure 9: Assessment of motivation to quit among surveyed smokers according to Q-MAT[d5]-_ score

- **Factors with a positive impact on motivation:**

A positive correlation was found between age (r=0.02), dependence (r =0.081), HAD score (depression: r=0.012, Anxiety: r= 0.2) and motivation to quit smoking. However, the relationship was negligible (r<0.2).

Among subjects with anxiety, 38% were highly motivated to quit smoking, 31% were moderately motivated, and 31% were insufficiently motivated.

The presence of a causal link between smoking and the pathology from which the hospitalized parent suffers seems to increase motivation to quit smoking (r=0.56) (Figure n°10). In fact, 43.4% of smokers with a parent treated for COPD, and 23.5% of those with a parent hospitalized for PBC, were highly motivated to stop smoking.

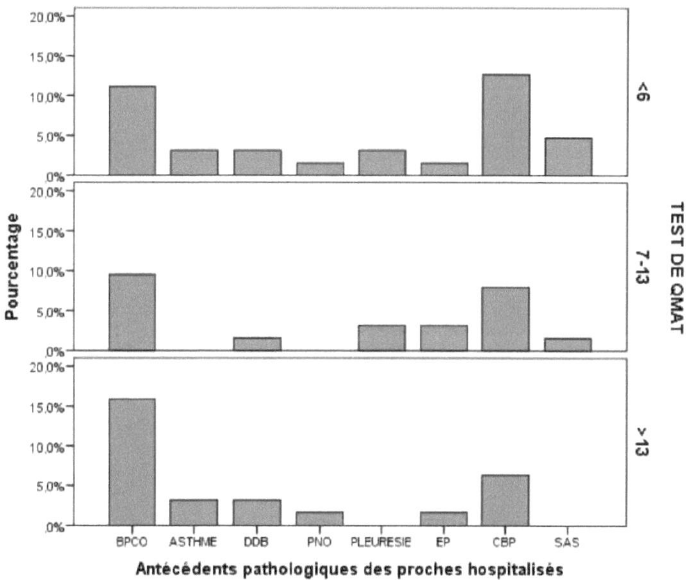

Figure 10: Motivation to quit smoking according to the pathology of the hospitalized parent.

DDB*: bronchial dilatation; PNO*: pneumothorax; PE*: pulmonary embolism; CBP*: bronchopulmonary cancer; SAS*: sleep apnea syndrome

- **Factors that have a negative impact on motivation:**

Low socio-economic status (r=-0.68), young age at first cigarette (r=-0.12), long duration of smoking (r=-0.003) and high PA consumption (r=-0.57) are associated with insufficient motivation to quit smoking.

The failure of previous attempts to quit smoking appears to have a negative influence on motivation to quit (r=-0.037).

9. IMPACT OF A LOVED ONE'S HOSPITALIZATION ON SMOKING CESSATION:

Fifteen percent (15%) of smokers surveyed had quit smoking at 3 months.

Among these subjects, 60% had a relative hospitalized for COPD decompensation and 20% had a relative being followed for PBC (figure n°11).

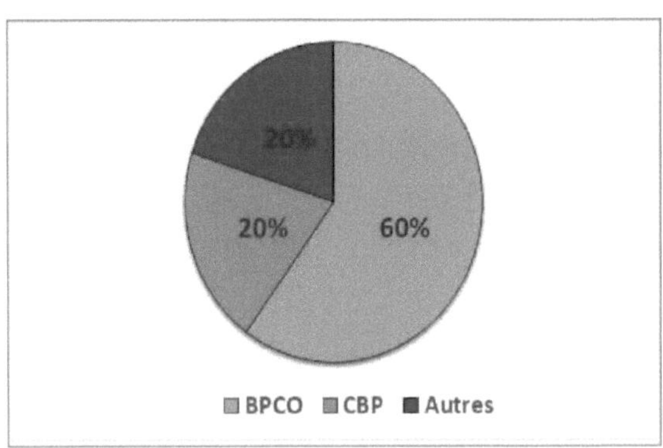

Figure 11: Percentage of subjects having quit smoking according to the pathology of their hospitalized relative.

A positive correlation was noted between smoking cessation at 3 months and tobacco dependence (p=0.039).

Discussion

1. EPIDEMIOLOGICAL DATA:

1.1. Prevalence:

1.1.1. Around the world:

More than a billion people worldwide continue to use tobacco products in 2017(12).

According to a new report by the World Health Organization (WHO), there has been a marked decline in smoking since 2000, but the reduction is insufficient to meet globally-agreed targets for avoiding death and suffering from cardiovascular and other non-communicable diseases (13).

For example, in Quebec, where smoking prevalence tends to be relatively high, the corresponding prevalence rates in 2014-2015 were 21% and 24% respectively (14).

1.1.2. In Tunisia:

Smoking prevalence in Tunisia was 24.9% in 2012 (15).

In 2016, according to the Ministry of Health, 23.5% of Tunisians were smokers: 45% of men, 3% of women and 20% of teenagers aged 11 and over.

1.2. Age:

Smoking has been described as a paediatric epidemic, with the majority of adult smokers starting in their teens (16).

The "Health behaviour in school-aged children (HBSC)" survey organized in 1997/1998 by the World Health Organization (WHO) in 31 countries around the world collected data from 123,227 adolescents aged 11, 13 and 15 respectively. Analysis of the data showed that tobacco experimentation increased with age in all countries and for both sexes. At age 11, around 20% of adolescents reported having tried smoking, at age 13 between 40 and 50%, and at age 15 between 60 and 70%(17).

In fact, despite a decline in prevalence, smoking remains highest among young adults aged 20 to 34.

In 2015 in Canada, 18.5% and 14.4% of young adults aged 20-24 and 25-34 respectively were smokers (18).

In our study, the average age of smokers was 40, with an average age of first smoking of 17.

1.3. Socioeconomic level:

Tobacco consumption rapidly leads to strong dependence, with a loss of control over the freedom not to smoke(19). The prevalence of smoking is higher among the poor. This behavior exacerbates their financial and health precariousness (20).

2. CHARACTERISTICS OF SMOKING:

2.1. Tobacco type:

Cigarettes dominate smoking patterns, and are more often associated with hookah among young people (21). Indeed, a Tunisian study involving 914 smokers from the general population found that young adults associated hookah much more with cigarettes (21).

This confirms the worrying scale of hookah consumption over the past decade (22).

In our study, cigarettes were the most commonly used type of tobacco (97% of cases versus 2.9% hookah consumption).

2.2. Duration and quantity of consumption:

Smoking needs to be accurately characterized (consumption, dependence, modalities and length of time) and, if possible, the rate of carbon monoxide poisoning needs to be measured (23).

Smoking-induced pathology is largely dependent on the number of cigarettes smoked, but it is the length of time smokers have been smoking that is most decisive in determining the risk of pathology.

Several authors have shown that the earlier the age at which smoking begins, the faster the transition to daily consumption (24-26).

A Tunisian study showed that young adults had earlier first experiences with tobacco, and became daily smokers more quickly. While older subjects showed greater physical dependence, consumed a greater number of cigarettes and had higher levels of carbon monoxide in exhaled air (COE) (21).

In our study, the average consumption was 28 BP, with 77% smoking more than 10 BP and 28% more than 30 BP, with an average smoking duration of 22 years.

3. TOBACCO AND RESPIRATORY DISEASES:

A meta-analysis including 216 articles highlighted the responsibility of active smoking in increasing the risk of COPD (RR = 4.01), asthma (RR = 1.61), bronchial cancer (RR = 10.92) and tuberculosis (27).

Furthermore, it is essential to identify smoking habits in all patients undergoing consultation for respiratory pathology. Between 38% and 77% of COPD sufferers continue to smoke (28). For bronchial cancer, doubling the dose doubles the risk, and doubling the duration of exposure multiplies the risk by 20 (29).

For the smokers interviewed in our study, no tobacco-related pathology was found.

4. TOBACCO ADDICTION:

Smoking is an addictive behavior combining psychobehavioral and pharmacological dimensions, in which nicotine, the main tobacco alkaloid, plays a key role, reinforced by the action of other monoamine oxidase inhibiting molecules present in tobacco smoke(30). Nicotine crosses the alveolar-capillary barrier as a free base, and within a few seconds reaches specific receptors on the brain's reward system (mesocortico-limbic), inducing a release of dopamine which is responsible for the sensation of satisfaction associated with inhalation (31).

The strength and speed of tobacco dependence are linked to the quantity of nicotine delivered and the speed with which it reaches the brain. In the absence of nicotine delivery, the addicted smoker experiences a withdrawal syndrome with "craving" (the need to consume a psychoactive substance (PAS) conditioned by the obsessive desire to enjoy it without delay)(32).

Physical dependence on tobacco, as assessed by the Fagerstrom score, is a prognostic factor for withdrawal failure (33-35).

In a Tunisian study carried out in 2015,the determinants of high smoking dependence were early age of first cigarette, duration of smoking, alcoholism, sedentary lifestyle and high WCC(21).

In our study, a positive correlation was found between age of first cigarette (p=0.02), number of APs (p=0.04) and tobacco dependence.

5. PSYCHOLOGICAL ASSESSMENT:

Identifying anxiety or depressive disorders is important, as they have an impact on withdrawal prognosis.

Shared vulnerability factors could explain the particular frequency of association between smoking and depression(36).

Several hypotheses have been put forward to explain the comorbidity of smoking and anxiety disorders, in particular the existence of tobacco-induced respiratory disorders and/or hypoxia intolerance (37).

An increase in suicidal risk proportional to the increase in cigarette consumption (never smoker: RR = 1, ex-smoker: RR = 1.4, smoker< 15 cigarettes per day (cigarette/d) = 2.6, smoker > 15cigarette/d = 4.5) has been demonstrated (38).

Emotional stress, often characterized by symptoms of anxiety and depression, has long been recognized as a major risk factor for relapse among smokers (39).

However, in the context of our work, is anxiety a motivating factor in smoking cessation? Indeed, a positive correlation was found between anxiety disorders and the pathology of the hospitalized relative. Subjects who had a close relative hospitalized for a tobacco-related pathology (chronic obstructive pulmonary disease, bronchopulmonary cancer) tended to have an anxiety disorder.

There was also a positive correlation between anxiety and motivation to quit smoking. Indeed, among subjects with anxiety, 38% were highly motivated to quit smoking, while 31% were moderately motivated.

6. MOTIVATION TO STOP SMOKING:

6.1. Assessment of motivation to stop smoking:

A French study carried out in 2008 investigated smoking cessation motivation using the QMAT in a male smoking population visiting a general practitioner. The study involved 32 subjects. In this study, 48% were insufficiently motivated, 32% moderately motivated and 19% strongly motivated (40).

In the USA, 68% of adults are smokers, but only 62% of 18-24 year-olds have expressed a desire to smoke (41).

In Canada, although over 62% of smokers aged 20-24 had tried to quit in the previous year, only 13% remained abstinent (18).

Young adults have difficulty quitting smoking partly because they don't use cessation programs, nicotine replacement therapy or other proven aids as much as older adults, preferring instead to quit without help (42, 43).

In our study, a strong motivation to quit smoking was observed in 32.9% of the subjects surveyed.

6.2. Factors influencing motivation to stop smoking:

6.2.1. Factors with a positive impact on motivation:

- **Managing anxiety:**

In the studies, the fight against stress came up in almost every interview as a justification for smoking. Tobacco was considered to have marked beneficial effects (calming, relaxation, anti-stress).

Other studies tend to prove that anxiety disorders most often appear after the onset of smoking(44). It also appears that smoking cessation can be accompanied by an improvement in anxiety(44).

This was the case for our study, given that a positive correlation was found between the presence of anxiety and the smoking-related respiratory pathology of the hospitalized relative. Indeed, these anxious subjects had relatives hospitalized for serious pathologies (COPD: 44% and PBC: 36.6%).

So it was an opportune moment to make these subjects aware of the harmful effects of smoking and encourage them to quit. It's the doctor's role to change this negative point (anxiety) and direct it towards a positive point (stopping smoking), by encouraging cessation to prevent the harmful effects of smoking.

It would therefore be very important to get this message across in weaning aid missions in these populations. We also need to take a holistic approach to the individual, and make the most of his or her living conditions to improve the chances of successful weaning.

- **Cigarette prices**

In the general population, the issue of cigarette prices was statistically responsible for 62.8% of smoking cessation (45). However, the very high level of dependence probably implied a continuation of smoking whatever the conditions (rolling tobacco, deeper inhalation, longer inspiratory pause, shorter butts) (45). In this way, they continue to absorb the same amount of nicotine with fewer cigarettes. Unfortunately, this procedure increases the quantity of toxic substances inhaled.

- **Smoking cessation aids:**

Lack of knowledge about smoking cessation aids and structures was often recognized as a barrier to cessation. This was compounded by a lack of confidence in the means of help. These items also recurred in the study population, especially concerning the unavailability and ineffectiveness of nicotine substitutes. Lack of knowledge about help structures was undoubtedly present as an obstacle to their cessation.

6.2.2. Factors that have a negative impact on motivation:

- **A socializing practice**

Smoking had often been initiated by peers or family at a very young age. Tobacco was an object of exchange, a socializing practice that created a strong bond. There was no shame in smoking, and the people around them were usually smokers.

In the general population, setting an example and the people around you were the most frequently cited reasons for quitting smoking.

- **Pleasure:**

Smoking was often referred to in the literature as "the last pleasure" (46). The people we interviewed did not emphasize this point. For them, smoking played a therapeutic and necessary role, rather than a pleasure.

- **Confidence in success:**

Studies have often shown that people have doubts about their own ability to stop smoking. Attempts to stop smoking are unlikely to lead to permanent cessation, and failure will further damage self-image.

- **Depressive syndrome:**

The links between smoking and depression are significant. As they probably share common genetic, psychological and behavioural vulnerability factors, patients wishing to stop smoking need to be monitored from a thymic point of view, especially if they are seeking help (47). The question of morale was addressed, as a depressive syndrome could have been an obstacle to proposing smoking cessation. Indeed, advising against smoking cessation because of depression reinforces the idea that many smokers are incapable of achieving anything, and worsens their depression(48).

Thus, a major depressive episode present at the start of cessation or occurring during cessation should be systematically sought. Its management should be presented as an integral part of the cessation aid, so as not to worsen the mood of the patient wishing to stop smoking(48).

7. Impact of a loved one's hospitalization on smoking cessation:

Fifteen percent of the subjects surveyed had quit smoking. It seems that answering the questionnaire is a motivating factor in quitting smoking. This reinforces the idea that cessation in these populations requires individualized, comprehensive care.

Motivational interviewing is an approach that effectively guides patients towards change. This collaborative, person-centred approach aims to explore, elicit and reinforce patients' motivation to change. Indeed, to be most effective, smoking cessation education should begin with minimal counseling and continue through an intensive smoking cessation program (49). Physicians can positively influence the ability of these subjects to quit smoking.

Galera et al suggest that an educational approach to smoking cessation is likely to help the majority of smoking patients to quit, without loss of morale or weight gain, and encourage the creation of a genuine therapeutic education program dedicated to smoking cessation (50).Some authors have determined that individual sessions of cognitive-behavioural therapy (CBT) increase the chances of successful smoking cessation by around 50%(51). This is one of the only non-medication approaches whose effectiveness has been scientifically demonstrated(51). Similarly, by intervening at a behavioral, cognitive and emotional level, CBTs aim to reduce relapse and encourage maintenance of smoking abstinence through new behavioral learning. They act on the behaviours that lead to smoking: self-taught programs, individual anti-smoking counselling, group therapies, self-help and social support groups and smoking habit modification techniques(52).

However, few of them integrate smoking cessation sessions into their routine practice. Prescribing NPTs could therefore help to achieve our goal of cessation in a variety of formats(53, 54).

The high nicotine dependency of our patients combined with the low uptake of nicotine replacement therapy and the absence of smoking cessation programs and legislation could explain the low success rate of smoking cessation.

The important thing is to take account of this difficulty in envisioning the future when setting up weaning support programs. Part of the support could be devoted to developing future projects.

Conclusion

Smoking is the leading preventable cause of death. Every year, it is responsible for over 6 million deaths worldwide. Tobacco consumption induces a dependency with genetic, pharmacological and environmental components. It is a chronic disease whose evolution is punctuated by attempts to quit and relapses.

We conducted a prospective, cross-sectional study over a 2-month period in 70 smokers with a relative hospitalized in the Sfax Pneumology Department. A questionnaire was administered to assess anxiety-depressive disorders (Hospital Anxiety and Depression Scale), physical dependence (Fagerstrom score) and motivation to stop smoking (Q-MAT scale). A telephone call was made at 3 months to reassess smoking status.

The 70 men had an average age of 40. The main type of tobacco used was filtered cigarettes (97%), followed by hookah (2.9%). The average age of the first cigarette was 17 years. The most frequent reasons for hospitalization of their relatives were COPD decompensation (36%) and bronchopulmonary cancer (27%). Average tobacco consumption was 29 PA. Dependence on tobacco was judged to be very severe (35.7%), moderate (18.6%), weak (20%) and absent (25.7%). A previous quit attempt was reported by 21.7% of subjects. Good motivation to quit smoking was found in 32.9% of cases. According to the HAD scale, anxiety disorders were noted in 41% of cases, and depressive disorders in 11%.

A positive association was noted between anxiety disorders and the cause of the parent's hospitalization. Indeed, subjects who had a relative hospitalized for a tobacco-related pathology (chronic obstructive pulmonary disease, bronchopulmonary cancer) tended to have an anxiety disorder. Among the anxious subjects surveyed, 44% had a relative hospitalized for COPD decompensation and 36.6% for PBC.

A positive correlation was found between age (r=0.02), dependence (r =0.081), HAD score (depression: r=0.012, Anxiety: r= 0.2) and motivation to quit smoking. However, the relationship was negligible (r<0.2).

Thirty-eight percent (38%) of anxious subjects surveyed were highly motivated to quit smoking, and 31% were moderately motivated.

The presence of a causal link between smoking and the pathology from which the hospitalized relative suffers seems to increase motivation to quit (r=0.56). Forty-three percent of smokers motivated to quit had relatives hospitalized for COPD and 23.5% for PBC.

After 3 months, 15% of smokers surveyed had quit. Among these subjects, 60% had a relative hospitalized for COPD decompensation and 20% had a relative being followed for PBC. A positive correlation was noted between smoking cessation at 3 months and tobacco dependence (p=0.039).

The study of their motivation to stop smoking revealed several areas of particular interest. It seems that stress linked to the pathology of a hospitalized loved one is a motivating factor. It is also important to note the high level of dependency and the difficulty of projecting oneself into the future, which are two obstacles to successful cessation. Smoking cessation aids need to take these particularities into account and offer a comprehensive approach. This should include work on stress, living conditions, future plans and self-esteem. This collaborative, person-centred approach is designed to explore, encourage and reinforce patients' motivation to change. In fact, to be most effective, smoking cessation education should begin with minimal counseling and continue through an intensive smoking cessation program.

We also need to take a holistic approach to the person concerned, and make the most of his or her living conditions to improve the chances of successful cessation. It's the doctor's role to change this negative point (anxiety) and steer it towards a positive point (stopping smoking), by encouraging cessation to prevent the harmful effects of smoking.

Bibliographies

1 **Jha P.Avoidable global cancer deaths and total deaths from smoking.**

Nature reviews Cancer. 2009;9(9):655-64.

2 **Eriksen M MJ, Schluger N, Islami F, Droppe J. The tobacco atlas. 5th Edition.**

Atlanta: American Thoracic Society. 2015;[Revised, expanded, and updated].

3 **Ribassin-Majed L, Hill C. Trends in tobacco-attributable mortality in France.**

European journal of public health. 2015;25(5):824-8.

4 **.Santé SodlOmdl. wwwwhoint/en.**

5 **Hughes JR, Keely J, Naud S. Shape of the relapse curve and long-term abstinence among untreated smokers.**

Addiction. 2004;99(1):29-38.

6 **Hanssens L, Lustygier V, Ansseau M, Thiebaut I, Thimpont J. [The motivational week: A new approach in smoking cessation].**

Journal of respiratory diseases. 2017;34(3):188-93.

7 **Lagrue G, Le Faou AL, Scemama O. [Smoking, the numbers need analysis].**

Presse medicale. 2005;34(15):1055-8.

8 **Perriot J. [Provision of smoking cessation therapy].**

Journal of Respiratory Diseases. 2006;23(1 Suppl):3S85-3S105.

9 Heatherton TF, Kozlowski LT, Frecker RC, Fagerstrom KO. **The Fagerstrom Test for Nicotine Dependence: a revision of the Fagerstrom Tolerance Questionnaire.**

British journal of addiction. 1991;86(9):1119-27.

10 **Aubin HJ LGLP, Azoulaï G, Pélisolo S, Humbert R, Renon D. Quit Smoking Motivation Questionnaire (Q-MAT).**

Alcohol Addictol. 2004;26:311-16.

11 . **Zigmond AS, Snaith RP. The hospital anxiety and depression scale.**

Acta psychiatrica Scandinavica. 1983;67(6):361-70.

12 .**OMdl Health. WHO report on the global tobacco epidemic, 2017** www.whoint/tobacco/global_report/2017/executive-summary/en/. 2017.

13 **Health OMdl. Smoking is declining, but too slowly. World No Tobacco Day: tobacco and heart disease.** 2018;

www.who.int/fr/news-room/detail/31-05-2018-world-no-tobacco-day-tobacco-and-heart- disease.

14 .**Institut de la statistique du Québec (2016). Enquête québécoise sur la santé de la population (EQSP) Quebec Population Health Survey 2016**

Available at: https://wwwinfocentreinspqrtssqcca (Retrieved March 19, 2017) 2014-2015.

15 **Jarraya F, Kammoun K, Mahfoudh H, Kammoun K, Hachicha J. [Management of arterial hypertension in Tunisia: the challenge of a developing country].**

Swiss Medical Journal. 2012;8(353):1725-6, 8-30.

16 Kessler DA, Witt AM, Barnett PS, Zeller MR, Natanblut SL, Wilkenfeld JP, et al. The Food and Drug Administration's regulation of tobacco products.

The New England journal of medicine. 1996;335(13):988-94.

17 .AGHAINN SN FY. Substance use. In Health and health behaviour among young people.

WHO Policy Series: Health policy for children and adolescents Issues. 2000;97-114.

18 .Reid JL, Hammond, D., Rynard, V. L., Madill, C. L., Burkhalter, R. Tobacco use in Canada: Patterns and trends (2017 Edition).

Waterloo, ON: Propel Centre for Population Health Impact, University of Waterloo Available at: wwwtobaccoreportca. 2017.

19 Ben Ayoub W DK, Stoebner-Delbarre A, Fakhfakh R, et al. La consultation d'aide au sevrage tabagique de l'institut de cancérologie Salah-Azeiz de Tunis: résultats à un an. Revue d'Épidémiologie et de Santé Publique. 2008;56:280-5.

20 Martinet Y WN, Béguinot E, Cagnat-Lardeau C. Tobacco control.

Jour Fran Viet Pul.02:6-13.

21 .Sriha Belguith Asma BI, Elmhamdi Sana, Ben Salah Aroua, Harizi Chahida, Ben Salem Kamel, Soltani Moahmed Essouss nicotine dependence and carbon monoxide intoxication in adult smokers.

La tunisie Medicale. 2015;Vol 93 (n°04):231-6.

22 Helmi Ben Saad. Hookah and its effects on health. Part II: the effects of hookah on health.2010;66:132-44.

23 **Wirth N PJ, Stoebner A, Peyrin-Biroulet C, TheveninC, Martinet Y. Tabagisme.**

In: La Pneumologie fondée sur lespreuves, sous l'égide de la SPLF, coordination S Marchand-Adam 5è édition Paris: Editions Margaux Orange. 2017.

24 **Hastier N, Quinque K, Bonnel AS, Lemenager S, Le Roux P. [Smoking and the adolescent. An inquiry into motivation and knowledge of the effects of tobacco].**

Journal of Respiratory Diseases. 2006;23(3 Pt 1):237-41.

25 **Hutchinson PJ, Richardson CG, Bottorff JL. Emergent cigarette smoking, correlations with depression and interest in cessation among Aboriginal adolescents in British Columbia.**

Canadian journal of public health = Revue canadienne de sante publique. 2008;99(5):418-22.

26 **Tavolacci MP, Marini H, Bailly L, Ladner J. [Prevalence and socio-health characteristic of hard-core smokers in Haute-Normandie].**

Sante publique. 2009;21(6):583-93.

27 **.Jayes L, Haslam PL, Gratziou CG, Powell P, Britton J, Vardavas C, et al. SmokeHaz: Systematic Reviews and Meta-analyses of the Effects of Smoking on Respiratory Health.** Chest. 2016;150(1):164-79.

28 **Tonnesen P. Smoking cessation and COPD.**

European respiratory review: an official journal of the European Respiratory Society. 2013;22(127):37-43.

29 **Hill C. [Tobacco epidemiology].**

La Revue du praticien. 2012;62(3):325, 7-9.

30 Perriot J, Underner M, Peiffer G, Dautzenberg B. [Helping smoking cessation in COPD, asthma, lung cancer, operated smokers].

Journal of clinical pulmonology. 2018;74(3):170-80.

31 Abrous N AH, Berlin I, Junien C, Kaminski M, Le Foll B, et al Tabac. Comprendre la dépendance pour agir.

Expertise collective Paris: Les Editions Inserm. 2004.

32 Brousse G CI. Craving: keys to understanding.

Alcohol Addictol. 2014; 36:105-15.

33 Li L, Borland R, Yong HH, Fong GT, Bansal-Travers M, Quah AC, et al. Predictors of smoking cessation among adult smokers in Malaysia and Thailand: findings from the International Tobacco Control Southeast Asia Survey.

Nicotine & tobacco research: official journal of the Society for Research on Nicotine and Tobacco. 2010;12 Suppl:S34-44.

34 .Sienkiewicz-Jarosz H, Zatorski P, Baranowska A, Ryglewicz D, Bienkowski P. Predictors of smoking abstinence after first-ever ischemic stroke: a 3-month follow-up. Stroke. 2009;40(7):2592-3.

35 Zhou X, Nonnemaker J, Sherrill B, Gilsenan AW, Coste F, West R. Attempts to quit smoking and relapse: factors associated with success or failure from the ATTEMPT cohort study.

Addictive behaviors. 2009;34(4):365-73.

36 Le Strat Y GP. Genetic vulnerabilities to smokingand anxiety, depression and psychoses.

In: Fédération franc, ai se de psychiatrie, Office franc,ais de prévention du tabagisme conférence d'experts, editors Arrêt du tabac chez lespatients atteints d'affections psychiatriques. 2009;Paris: OFT Entre-prise.

37 Moylan S, Jacka FN, Pasco JA, Berk M. How cigarette smoking may increase the risk of anxiety symptoms and anxiety disorders: a critical review of biological pathways. Brain and behavior. 2013;3(3):302-26.

38 Miller M HD, Rimm E. Cigarette and suicide:a prospective study of 50,000 men.

Am J Public Health. 2000;90:768-73

39 .Cohen S, Lichtenstein E. Perceived stress, quitting smoking, and smoking relapse.

Health psychology: official journal of the Division of Health Psychology, American Psychological Association. 1990;9(4):466-78.

40 .N NG. Intérêt du dépistage de la dysfonction érectile dans la motivation au cessage tabagique: à propos d'une enquête en médecine générale [Thèse d'exercice].

[France]: Université Paul Sabatier(Toulouse) Faculté des sciences médicales Rangueil; 2008.

41 .US Department of Health and Human Services. The health consequences of smoking- 50 years of progress: A report of the surgeon general.

Atlanta: US Department of Health and Human Services, Centers for Disease Control and Prevention, National Center for Chronic Disease Prevention and Health Promotion, Office on Smoking and Health 2014.

42 Solberg LI, Boyle RG, McCarty M, Asche SE, Thoele MJ. **Young adult smokers: are they different?** The American journal of managed care. 2007;13(11):626-32.

43 .Curry SJ, Sporer AK, Pugach O, Campbell RT, Emery S. Use of tobacco cessation treatments among young adult smokers: 2005 National Health Interview Survey.

Am J Public Health. 2007;97(8):1464-9.

44 Santé HAd. Therapeutic strategies for smoking cessation.

Effectiveness, efficiency and financial management. 2007.

45 Craig L GR, Wilquin J-L, Beck F, Arwidson P, Deutsch A, et al. ITC France National Report: Results of the second wave. Promoting evidence-based strategies to counter the global tobacco epidemic.

Waterloo (CAN): University of Waterloo 2011.

46 Constance J P-WP La cigarette du pauvre. Ethnologie française. 2010;40(3):535-42.

47 Lagrue G, Dupont P, Fakhfakh R. [Anxiety and depressive disorders in tobacco dependence]. L'Encephale. 2002;28(4):374-7.

48 .P. DUPONT SdAdPR, CHU Paul Brousse, VILLEJUIF. Depression and smoking cessation.

Practical information on tobacco.

49 .Smith PM, Burgess E. Smoking cessation initiated during hospital stay for patients with coronary artery disease: a randomized controlled trial.

CMAJ: Canadian Medical Association journal = journal de l'Association medicale canadienne. 2009;180(13):1297-303.

50 .O. Galeraa DB, Z. Maoza, C. Lussagneta, Tadiotto, T. Babina. Effectiveness of therapeutic education against "nicotinophobia" in patientssmokers hospitalized in cardiovascular and pulmonary follow-up and rehabilitation care.

Journal of clinical pulmonology. 2017;5.

51.Lancaster T, Stead LF. Individual behavioural counselling for smoking cessation.

The Cochrane database of systematic reviews. 2017;3:CD001292.

52 Smoking cessation.

Référentiels Auvergne-Rhône-Alpes en oncologie thoracique, 10th Edition Updated 2016.

53 Meine TJ, Patel MR, Washam JB, Pappas PA, Jollis JG. Safety and effectiveness of transdermal nicotine patch in smokers admitted with acute coronary syndromes.

The American journal of cardiology. 2005;95(8):976-8.

54 Guevel-Jointret AL, Borel ML, Munier S, Cornily JC, Pennec PY, Gilard M, et al [Tolerance and efficacy of early nicotine substitution after acute coronary syndromes].

Archives of Heart and Vascular Diseases. 2007;100(6-7):514-8.

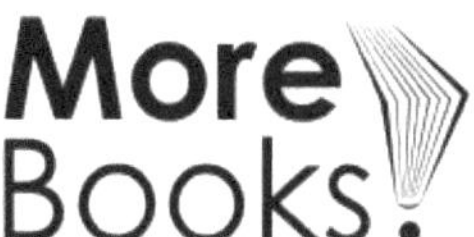

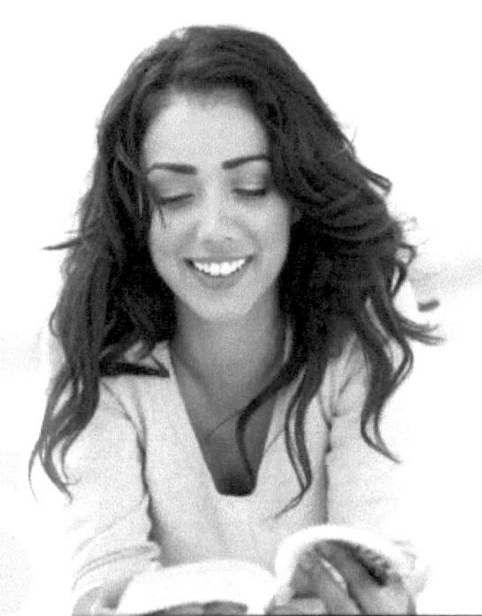

I want morebooks!

Buy your books fast and straightforward online - at one of world's fastest growing online book stores! Environmentally sound due to Print-on-Demand technologies.

Buy your books online at
www.morebooks.shop

Kaufen Sie Ihre Bücher schnell und unkompliziert online – auf einer der am schnellsten wachsenden Buchhandelsplattformen weltweit! Dank Print-On-Demand umwelt- und ressourcenschonend produziert.

Bücher schneller online kaufen
www.morebooks.shop

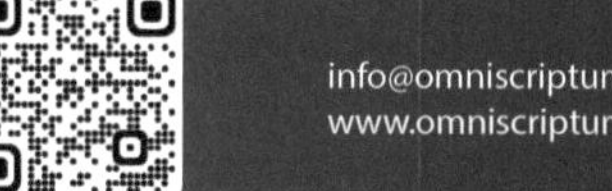

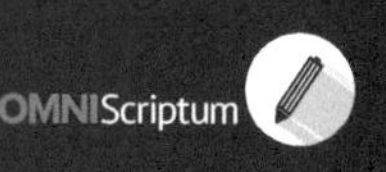

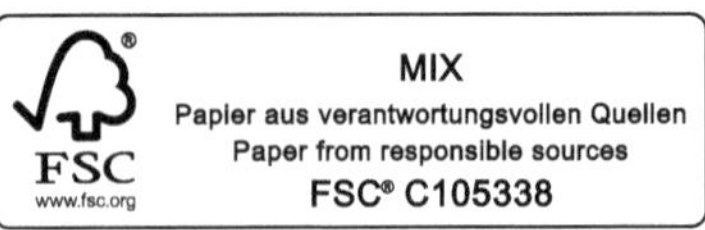

Printed by Books on Demand GmbH, Norderstedt / Germany